THE LITTLE RED BOOK OF ACUPUNCTURE

A handbook of control points of the meridians and
rules of the circulation of energy.

THE LITTLE RED BOOK OF ACUPUNCTURE

by

Dr J.P. LEGER

Member of the Association Scientifique des Médicins Acupuncteurs de France

Translated from the French by
Geoffrey A. Dudley, B.A.

NATURE'S WAY

THORSONS PUBLISHERS LIMITED
Wellingborough, Northamptonshire

Published in France as *le petit livre
rouge de l'acupuncture*
© Maloine S.A. Editeur, Paris, 1976
First published in England 1978

© THORSONS PUBLISHERS LIMITED 1978

ISBN 0 7225 0430 6

Photoset in Great Britain by
Specialised Offset Services Limited, Liverpool
and printed by
Weatherby Woolnough, Wellingborough, Northamptonshire

DEDICATION

To Dr R. Casez
who explained so well the subtle
game of the regulation of energy
at a minor Congress at Lyons in
1962.

CONTENTS

FOREWORD

Dr Léger and I first got to know each other at the *Ecole Principale du Service de Santé de la Marine et des Troupes de Marine*, and then later, much later, we were both acupuncturists – one more reason for keeping in touch. Like all of us, he has 'knocked about in the tropics' for more than thirty years, twenty of which were spent in the Far East, observing, studying, inquiring into everything around him.

So it was that, one day in 1939, the Marine Light Infantry Colonel in command of the *Marsouins*[1] of the French concession of Hue, who was a well-informed scholar and expert in the Chinese language, spoke to him about his high blood-pressure, which was over 200. He politely rejected any treatment by orthodox practitioners, saying to him simply: 'Let's go to Quang Ngai to see old Luong.' And there, 125 miles away, he saw, not without astonishment, old Luong insert some needles into the Colonel's wrists – and the latter's blood-pressure dropped to 160.

What might have remained only an episode of folklore became a subject of close study when, during a short stay in France in 1947, Dr Léger's father, a doctor like himself, gave him G. Soulié de Morant's *Précis de la vraie acupuncture chinoise* to read.

[1] A nickname for French colonial infantry troops. – *Trans.*

This work, which is an excellent starting-point for the study of the traditional art of medicine with its rules of the circulation of energy, was the basis of instruction in acupuncture by the *Société d'Acupuncture* and has remained so for the *Association Scientifique des Médecins Acupuncteurs de France*, which today continues to work to the same effect.

That is why, considering that the explanations by the longer works are sometimes involved, confused, and often tedious for beginners who have no one by their side to direct their studies, Dr Léger has aimed to present the general rules of Chinese energizing medicine and their application in the form of a clear, practical summary in a small format which would be easy to refer to.

Like him, may his *Little Red Book* contrive to go into different corners of the world and present to those who are drawn to acupuncture the bases of the ancient traditional medicine which the ASMAF continues to pursue by striving to unravel its mysteries through modern scientific research.

Dr GEORGES GRALL
Vice-President of the ASMAF and
Director of Studies

PREFACE

Thirty years ago very few practitioners of acupuncture existed in the west, but today their number has grown considerably, and more and more interest is being shown both by lay people and the orthodox medical profession. The ancient science is being vindicated by modern research and with the development of new techniques there has arisen a 'neo-acupuncture'. But, although there are many new techniques, the time-honoured classical theory of the *circulation of energy*, which for centuries has enabled spectacular results to be obtained, still remains the very essence of acupuncture.

For the successful diagnosis of complaints it is necessary to be able to accurately read the pulses, and to do this practitioners must have a sound knowledge of the control points of the meridians as well as the points of common action, and the rules of the circulation of energy and of reciprocal effects. To obtain this knowledge it is generally necessary to study the many and voluminous classical works on the subject, and the purpose of this book is to gather together, with purely pragmatic goals, what is scattered, so as to facilitate the work of students and practitioners.

To simplify things, the questions of the five elements, the deep circulation and Yin and Yang have been put aside and the emphasis has been put on the distribution of energy among the meridians.

The points studied consist of: 1. The circulation of energy; 2. The pulses and their interpretation; 3. The control points of the meridians; 4. The points of common action on several meridians; 5. The rules of reciprocal action and the technique of the regulation of energy.

LIST OF SYMBOLS AND ABBREVIATIONS

—————	– Yang Meridians
—–—–—	– Yin Meridians
—➤——	– Direction of the circulation
B	– Bladder
D	– Dispersion Point
Ent	– Entry Point
Ex	– Exit Point
GB	– Gall-bladder
H	– Heart
h	– High
Her	– Herald Point
JM	– Jen-Mo Meridian (Conception Vessel)
K	– Kidney
L	– Luo Point
l	– Low
LI	– Large Intestine
Lu	– Lung
Lv	– Liver
P	– Pericardium
S	– Stomach
SI	– Small Intestine
So	– Source Point
SP	– Spleen – Pancreas
T	– Tonification Point
TM	– Tu-Mo Meridian (Governing Vessel)
TW	– Triple Warmer

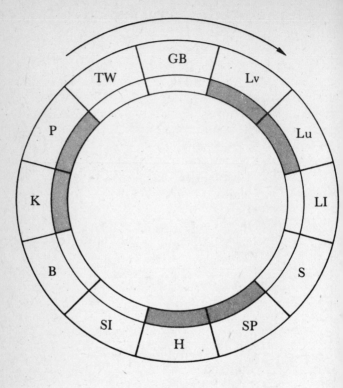

Figure 1
Diagram of the circulation of energy

CHAPTER ONE

THE CIRCULATION OF ENERGY

Acupuncture points, with the exception of those of the ear and isolated ones called 'extraneous points and neo-acupuncture points', the connections of which are still not well known, are located along the paths of the fourteen meridians, which are presented as channels or lines of force on which energy circulates and travels through the body.

This circulation passes from one meridian into another, each communicating freely with the one that precedes it and the one that follows it. It should be noted, however, that this flow does not always take place end to end by intercommunication, but often by points well away from their extremity. This is why energy enters the meridian of the large intestine by its point No. 4, and leaves that of the gall-bladder by its point No. 41, whereas the meridian terminates at point No. 44.

If one excludes the axial meridians of Jen-Mo and Tu-Mo, which form a special network and of which the energy cannot be assessed by the pulses, the circulation occurs in a definite and uniform order known as the circuit of the circulation of energy.

Let us suppose that we are starting from the meridian of the gall-bladder: energy leaves this meridian in order to pass into that of the liver, then into that of the lung, the large intestine, the stomach, the spleen-pancreas, heart, small intestine, bladder, kidney, pericardium, triple warmer, and the circuit closes again at the gallbladder.

This cycle is objectified by a circle called 'Circuit of the main circulation of energy' (Figure 1).

It is conceivable that if an obstacle arises in this circuit, everything that lies upsteam will develop an excess and everything that lies downstream a shortage of energy. For the Chinese, this obstacle is the true origin of disease, and the acupuncturist's role is to raise this obstacle by stimulating the appropriate point or points.

CHAPTER TWO

THE PULSES AND THEIR INTERPRETATION

Inequality of energy in certain meridians is the expression of a pathological condition. Hence it is important to try to locate where the meridians with excess or shortage of energy are. This diagnosis is established by taking the Chinese pulses.

The table in Figure 2 represents the pulses of the meridians at their sites in the right and left wrists. For greater clarity, the deep Yin pulses have been displaced outwards and shaded.

Two pulses superimposed on the same anatomical site, such as GB and Lv, are said to be coupled. Two symmetrical pulses on the same level are called husband-wife – for example, Lu and H.

Examination of the radial pulses gives us a subjective idea of the quantity of energy which each meridian contains in relation to the others. So it is necessary to ascertain from these where the excesses and shortages of energy are and assess that value.

The standard authors praise the pulses with a marvellous range of epithets in which flights of poetic fancy contend with folklore. Our aim being to determine whether the circulation of energy is disturbed, in which case action must be taken, we shall content ourselves with noting the value of each pulse compared with the others by allotting 0 to 1 to very weak pulses that need strengthening and 4 or 5 to those with an excess that needs dispersing.

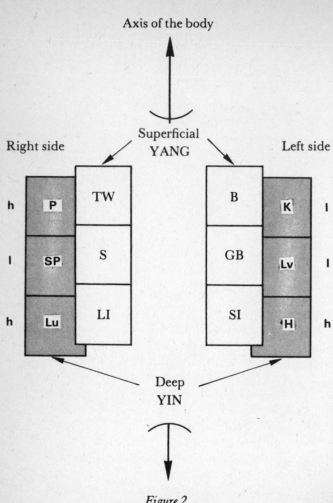

Axis of the body

Right side

Superficial
YANG

Left side

h	P	TW		B	K	l
l	SP	S		GB	Lv	l
h	Lu	LI		SI	H	h

Deep
YIN

Figure 2
Table of the pulses

18

CHAPTER THREE

THE CONTROL POINTS OF THE MERIDIANS

The control points of the meridians can be classed in two categories:

1st category. These are the points which act only in a given direction on the energizing level of the meridian, regardless of the tonifying or dispersing technique of insertion of the needle.

Two of these points raise the energy level of the meridian: 1. The point of tonification; 2. The herald point; and two lower the energy level: 3. The point of dispersion; 4. The point of assent.

2nd category. Depending on the stimulation applied to them (tonifying or dispersing), these points can raise or lower the energizing level of the meridian. They are: 5. The Luo points; 6. The source points; 7. The points of entry and exit.

The first category of these points plays the role of valves, allowing the energizing current to pass only in a given direction: towards the meridian for the herald points and points of tonification, away from the meridian for the points of dispersion and assent – regardless of the tonifying or dispersing technique of the insertion.

The points of the second category play a bypass role, allowing the current to pass only in the direction laid down by the technique of insertion.

Entry	Lu/1 Chong Fu	On the 2nd rib, 2 inches inside the axillary[1] line.
Tonification	Lu/9 Tai Yuan	At the intersection of the radial artery and the fold of the wrist.
Herald	Lu/1 Chong Fu	
Source	Lu/9 Tai Yuan	
Luo	Lu/7 Lie Tsiu	On the radial artery 2 inches above the fold of the wrist, 0.15 of the distance Lu/9 to Lu/5.
Dispersion	Lu/5 Chi Tse	At the bend of the elbow, on the outer edge of the tendon of the biceps.
Assent	B/13 Fei Yu	Paravertebral line below the apophysis of the 8th dorsal vertebra.
Exit	Lu/7 Lie Tsiu	

[1] Medical and other terms used in this book are defined in the Glossary (page 63). – *Trans.*

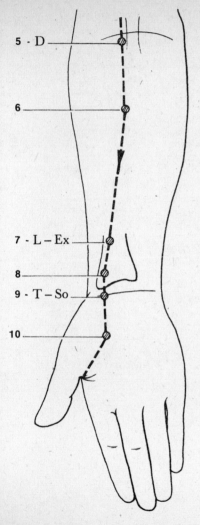
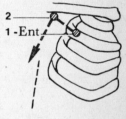

5 · D

6

7 · L – Ex

8

9 · T – So

10

2

1 · Ent

PERICARDIUM

Entry	P/1 Tien Chi	Under the 4th rib, 1 inch outside the nipple.
Tonification	P/9 Tshong Chong	1/12 inch behind the outer corner of the nail of the middle finger.
Herald	Not known	
Source	P/7 Ta Ling	In the centre of the bend of the wrist.
Luo	P/6 Nei Koan	2 inches above P/7, or 1/5 of the distance from the centre of the fold of the wrist to the centre of the bend of the elbow.
Dispersion	P/7 Ta Ling	
Assent	B/14 Tsiu Yin Yu	Paravertebral line under the spinous apophysis of the 4th dorsal vertebra.
Exit	P/8 Lao Kong	Flat of the hand, in the centre of the 3rd intermetacarpal space.

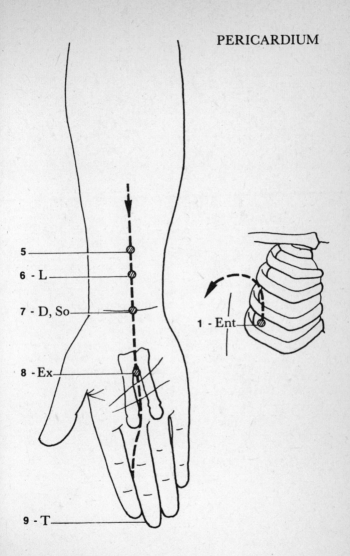

5

6 - L

7 - D, So

8 - Ex

9 - T

1 - Ent

HEART

Entry	H/1 Tsi Tsiuan	Under the 3rd rib, 1 inch inside the axillary line.
Tonification	H/9 Shao Chong	1/12 inch behind the corner of the nail of the little finger, ring-finger side.
Herald	JM/14 Tsiu Koan	¼ of the distance from the tip of the xiphoid appendage to the navel.
Source	H/7 Shen Men	At the juncture of the line bisecting the angle formed by the fold of the wrist and the cubital edge of the hand with the infero-external edge of the pisiform bone.
Luo	H/5 Tong Li	At the point of the styloid apophysis of the cubitus.
Assent	B/15 Sin Yu	Paravertebral line under the spinous aophysis of the 5th dorsal vertebra.
Dispersion	H/7 Shen Men	
Exit	H/9 Shao Chong	

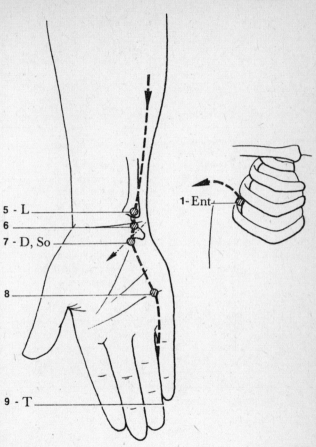

5 - L

6

7 - D, So

8

1- Ent

9 - T

LARGE INTESTINE

Entry	LI/4 Ro Ku	At the apex of the angle formed by the first two metacarpals.
Tonification	LI/11 Isiu Chi	At the outer extremity of the bend of the elbow.
Herald	S/25 Tien Chu	On the horizontal line of the navel, 3 inches outside it.
Source	LI/4 Ro Ku	
Luo	LI/6 Pien Li	Palm of the hand downward, on the outer edge of the radius, 0.3 of the distance from the fold of the wrist to the epicondyle.
Dispersion	LI/2 El Tsien	At the outer extremity of the bend of the index finger, on the palm.
Assent	B/25 Tao Chong Yu	Paravertebral line under the spinous pophysis of the 4th lumbar vertebra.
Exit	LI/20 Ying Siang	Above the bulge of the alae of the nose.

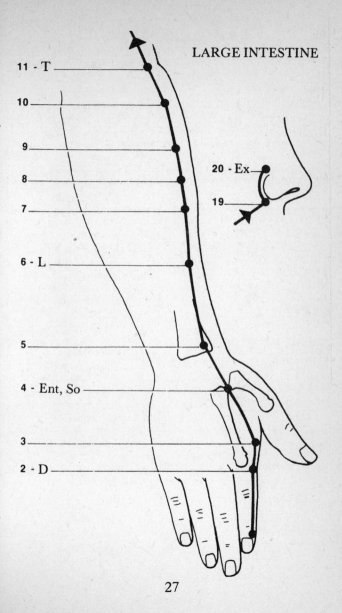

LARGE INTESTINE

11 - T
10
9
8
7
6 - L
5
4 - Ent, So
3
2 - D

20 - Ex
19

27

Entry	TW/1 Koan Chong	1/12 inch behind the corner of the nail of the ring-finger, on the side towards the little finger.
Tonification	TW/3 Chong Chu	At the apex of the angle formed by the 4th and 5th metacarpals.
Herald	JM/5 Shi Men	2/5 of the distance from the navel to the upper edge of the pubis.
Source	TW/4 Yang Chi	In the centre of the dorsal bend of the wrist.
Luo	TW/5 Wai Koan	Forearm bent back, hand on the shoulder, 1/5 of the distance from the dorsal bend of the wrist to the olecranon.
Dispersion	TW/10 Tien Tsing	At the apex of the olecranon, arm extended.
Assent	B/22 San Tsiao Yu	Paravertebral line under the spinous apophysis of the 1st lumbar vertebra.
Exit	TW/23 El Men	In the hollow above the tragus.

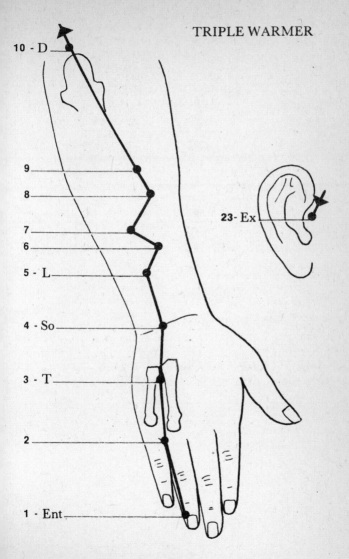

10 - D

9

8

7

6

5 - L

4 - So

3 - T

2

1 - Ent

23 - Ex

SMALL INTESTINE

Entry	SI/1 Shao Tse	1/12 inch behind the corner of the nail of the little finger, on the cubitus side.
Tonification	SI/3 Hou Tsi	At the cubital extremity of the fold of the palm.
Herald	JM/4 Koan Yuan	3/5 of the distance from the navel to the upper edge of the pubis.
Source	SI/4 Wan Ku	Tip of the unciform bone.
Luo	SI/7 Tshi Tsheng	Midway between the styloid apophysis and the bend of the elbow.
Dispersion	SI/8 Siao Hai	In the epitrochlear groove, elbow bent.
Assent	B/27 Sia Chang Yu	1 inch outside the 1st sacral fossa.
Exit	SI/18 Tsiuan Tsiao	In the angle of the zygoma and the ascending branch of the cheek-bone.

SMALL INTESTINE

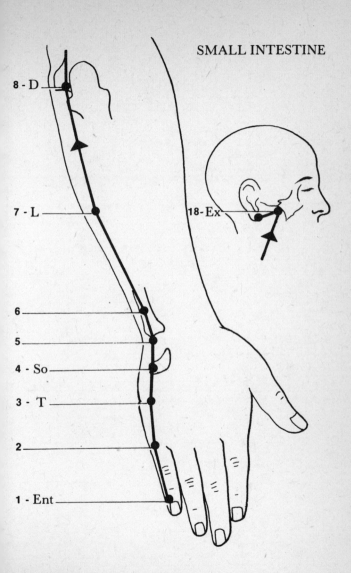

8 - D

7 - L

6

5

4 - So

3 - T

2

1 - Ent

18 - Ex

LIVER

Entry	Lv/2 Sing Tsien	At the extremity of the small fold formed by the 1st space between the toes, and going towards the big toe.
Tonification	Lv/8 Tsiu Tsiuan	At the inner extremity of the bend of the knee.
Herald	Lv/14 Tsi Men	Inder the 5th rib, outside the line of the nipple and 1 inch from it.
Source	Lv/3 Tai Chong	At the apex of the angle formed by the first two metatarsal bones.
Luo	Lv/5 Li Kou	Inner surface of the tibia, at 5/14 of the distance from the internal malleolus of the anterior prominence of the tibia.
Dispersion	Lv/2 Sing Tsien	
Assent	B/18 Kan Yu	Paravertebral line under the spinous apophysis of the 8th dorsal vertebra.
Exit	Lv/14 Tsi Men	

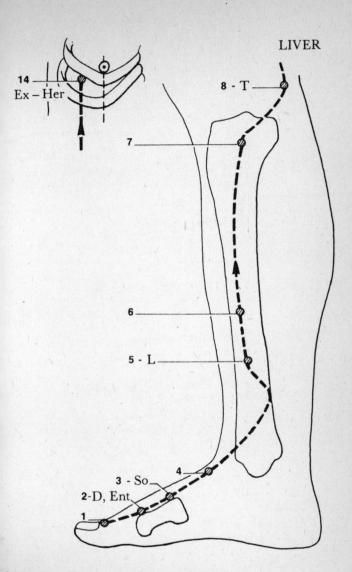

LIVER

14
Ex – Her

8 - T

7

6

5 - L

4

3 - So
2-D, Ent
1

SPLEEN – PANCREAS

Entry	SP/1 Yin Po	1/12 inch behind the inner corner of the nail of the big toe.
Tonification	SP/2 Ta Tu	Inside edge of the foot, in the hollow at the base of the metatarso-phalangeal joint.
Herald	Lv/13 Tshang Men	Under the 10th rib, level with the extremity of the 11th.
Source	SP/3 Tai Po	Behind and below the anterior extremity of the 1st metatarsal.
Luo	SP/4 Kong Sun	Under the 1st tarso-metatarsal joint.
Dispersion	SP/5 Shang Tsiu	Subject standing, at the juncture of a horizontal line passing through the tip of the internal malleolus and a vertical line passing through the centre of the tubercle of the scaphoid bone.
Assent	B/20 Pi Yu	Paravertebral line, under the apophysis of the 11th dorsal vertebra.
Exit	SP/21 Ta Pao	Under the 7th rib, on the anterior axillary line.

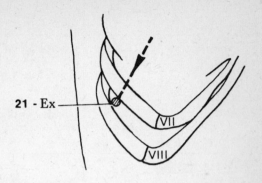

21 - Ex

VII

VIII

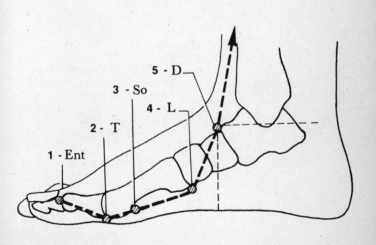

5 - D

3 - So

4 - L

2 - T

1 - Ent

KIDNEY

Entry	K/1 Yong Tsiuan	Anterior part of the sole of the foot, at the point where the creases meet
Tonification	K/7 Fu Liu	2 inches behind the posterior edge of the tibia and 2½ inches above the internal malleolus.
Herald	GB/25 Tsing Men	Lower edge of the 10th rib, on the anterior axillary line.
Source	K/3 Tai Tsi	1 inch behind the internal malleolus, on the upper edge of the heel-bone.
Luo	K/4 Ta Tshong	At the insertion of the Achilles tendon on the heel-bone.
Dispersion	K/1 Yong Tsiuan	
Assent	B/23 Shen Yu	Paravertebral line under the spinous apophysis of the 2nd lumbar vertebra.
Exit	K/22 Pu Lang	At the anterior extremity of the 5th intercostal space.

KIDNEY

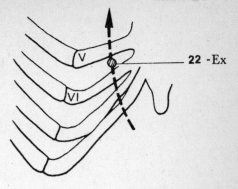

V

VI

22 -Ex

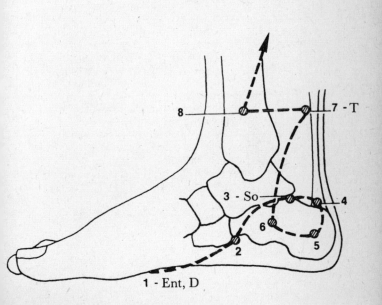

8

7 - T

3 - So

4

6

5

2

1 - Ent, D

BLADDER

Entry	B/1 Tsing Ming	1/12 inch inside the inner corner of the eyelid.
Tonification	B/67 Tshi Yin	1/12 inch behind the outer corner of the nail of the little toe.
Herald	JM/3 Tshong Tsi	1/5 of the distance from the upper edge of the pubis to the navel.
Source	B/64 Tsing Ku	Behind and below the protuberance of the 5th metatarsal bone.
Luo	B/58 Fei Yang	In the centre of the posterior edge of the fibula.
Dispersion	B/65 Shu Ku	Under the anterior extremity of the 5th metatarsal bone.
Assent	B/28 Pang Koang Yu	1 inch outside the 2nd sacral fossa.
Exit	B/67 Tshi Yin	

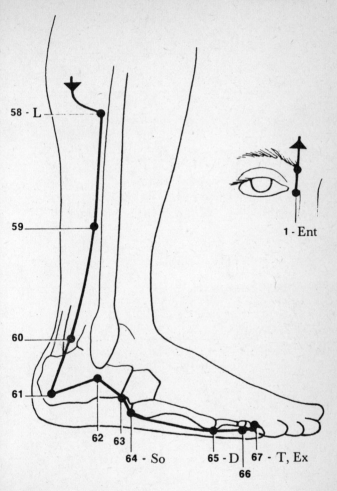

58 - L

59

60

61

62   63

64 - So

65 - D

66

67 - T, Ex

1 - Ent

Entry	GB/1 Tong Tsi Tsiao	1 inch outside the rim of the eye socket, on the upper edge of the zygoma.
Tonification	GB/43 Sia Tsi	At the base of the 4th toe, outer side.
Herald	GB/24 Ji Yue	On the chest, arms at sides, lower edge of the 6th rib on a vertical line 1 inch outside the nipple.
Source	GB/40 Tsiu Siu	Anterior outer surface of the foot, in the centre of the calcaneo-cuboid joint.
Luo	GB/37 Koang Ming	Anterior edge of the fibula, 4 inches above the malleolus.
Dispersion	GB/38 Yang Fu	Anterior edge of the fibula, 3 inches above the malleolus.
Assent	B/10 Tan Yu	Paravertebral line, below the spinous apophysis of the 9th dorsal vertebra.
Exit	GB/41 Lin Tsi	At the apex of the gap between the proximal extremities of the 4th and 5th metatarsal bones.

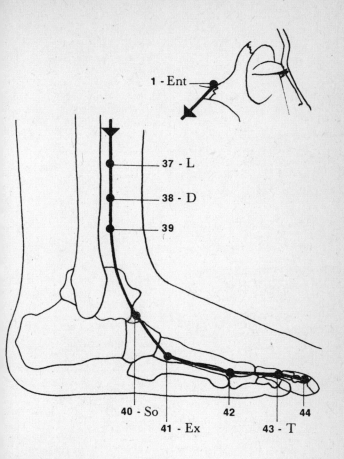

1 - Ent

37 - L

38 - D

39

40 - So

41 - Ex

42

43 - T

44

STOMACH

Entry	S/1 Tou Wei	1¼ inches above the tip of the eyebrow.
Tonification	S/41 Tsia Tsi	In the centre of the front of the ankle, in the depression below the tibia.
Herald	JM/12 Tshong Koan	Midway between the sternum and the navel, excluding the xiphoid appendage.
Source	S/42 Chong Lang	Bridge of the foot, at the junction of the scaphoid bone and the 2nd and 3rd cuneiform bones.
Luo	S/40 Fong Long	Anterior edge of the fibula, 1 inch above the centre of the line going from the external malleolus to the anterior protuberance of the tibia.
Dispersion	S/45 Li Tui	1/12 inch behind the outer corner of the nail of the 2nd toe.
Assent	B/21 Wei Yu	Paravertebral line under the spinous apophysis of the 12th dorsal vertebra.
Exit	S/42 Chong Lang	

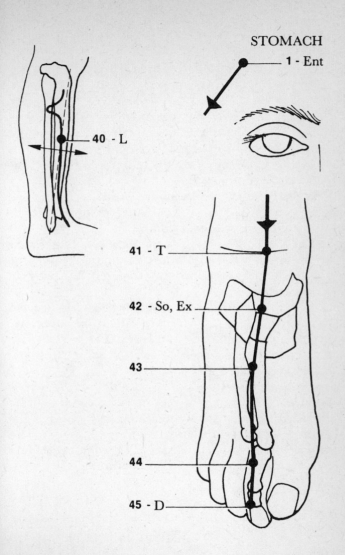

STOMACH

1 - Ent

40 - L

41 - T

42 - So, Ex

43

44

45 - D

THE HERALD POINTS

So as not to clutter the line drawings of the control points of the meridians, the herald points have not been included: they are shown separately here.

They are all found on the anterior surface of the chest and abdomen.

A sharp pain produced by pressure applied to their site indicates a functional disorder of the organ affected by the meridian.

They are used as a contributory invigorating stimulus in the regulation of energy, and the needles must therefore be inserted by way of tonification.

To tonify: The tip of the needle must be directed towards the exit point of a meridian by successive stages during inhalation, turning it in a clockwise direction. It must then be left for some time and withdrawn in a single movement.

To disperse: Insert the needle in a single movement, turning it counter-clockwise during exhalation, with the tip of the needle towards the point of entry of the meridian.

If possible, tonification should be done with gold needles, and dispersion with silver ones.

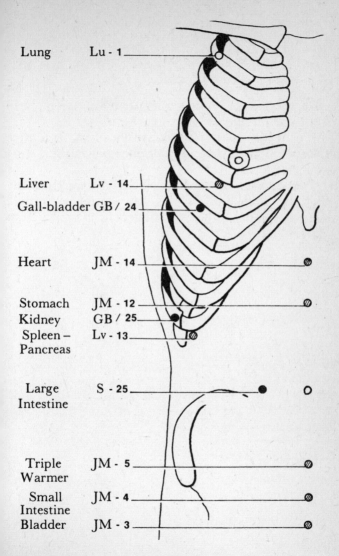

Lung — Lu - 1

Liver — Lv - 14
Gall-bladder GB / 24

Heart — JM - 14

Stomach — JM - 12
Kidney — GB / 25
Spleen – — Lv - 13
Pancreas

Large — S - 25
Intestine

Triple — JM - 5
Warmer
Small — JM - 4
Intestine
Bladder — JM - 3

THE POINTS OF ASSENT

Like the herald points, the points of assent have been shown together in a separate diagram.

Their stimulation has a sedative and regulative effect, which is used as a complement to the points of dispersion.

The points of assent are all located on the bladder meridian in its paravertebral dorsal branch, the breadth of two fingers or $1\frac{1}{2}$ inches from the spinal cord.

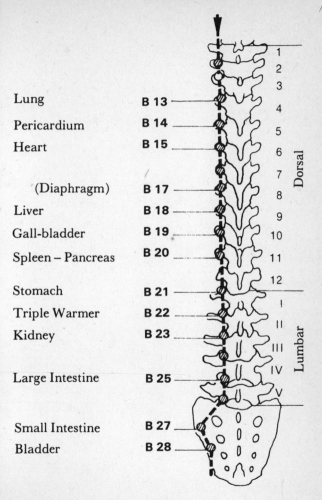

Lung	**B 13**	1 2 3 4
Pericardium	**B 14**	5
Heart	**B 15**	6
		7
(Diaphragm)	**B 17**	8
Liver	**B 18**	9
Gall-bladder	**B 19**	10
Spleen – Pancreas	**B 20**	11
		12
Stomach	**B 21**	I
Triple Warmer	**B 22**	II
Kidney	**B 23**	III
		IV
Large Intestine	**B 25**	V
Small Intestine	**B 27**	
Bladder	**B 28**	

Dorsal

Lumbar

CHAPTER FOUR

THE POINTS OF COMMON ACTION ON SEVERAL MERIDIANS

Some points act directly on several meridians at the same time. When the needles are inserted for tonification, these points strengthen the meridians which they connect; their dispersion acts in the opposite direction on the same meridians.

Of these common-action points, only the two categories which are the most useful in practice are mentioned, so as not to go beyond the pragmatic purpose of this work. They are the *group Luo* points and certain *ordinary centre-reunion* points.

THE GROUP LUO POINTS

Depending on the technique employed (invigorative or sedative), these control three adjoining meridians: Yan of the upper limp, Yin of the upper limb, Yang of the lower limb, Yin of the lower limb.

TW/8 San Yang Lo	Dorsal surface of the forearm, 4 inches from the cubital styloid.	Controls the Yangs Si, LI, TW
P/5 Tshien Shi	Anterior surface of the forearm, 4 inches above the centre of the bend of the wrist.	Controls the Yins of the arm. Lu, P H
GB/39 Siuan Tshong	Anterior edge of the fibula, 2 inches above the external malleolus.	Controls the Yangs of the leg. B, GB, S
SP/6 San Yin Tsiao	On the inner edge of the tibia, 3/14 of the distance from the tip of the internal malleolus to the anterior protuberance of the tibia.	Controls the Yins of the leg. K, Lv, SP

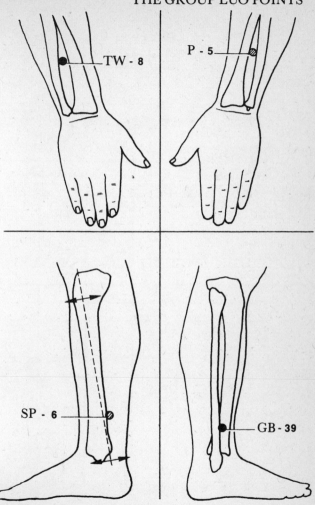

TW - 8

P - 5

SP - 6

GB - 39

THE ORDINARY CENTRE-REUNION POINTS

These points have the property of acting upon several meridians at the same time, including Jen-Mo and Tu-Mo. Their number is considerable, but, because some of them have identical properties while others affect only one meridian besides those

| Points for insertion | Meridians | | | | | |
| | YIN | | | | | |
	H	P	Lu	Lv	SP	K
S/1						
S/6						
S/12			+			
SI/12						
SI/18						
B/1						
B/11			+	+	+	
B/33						
GB/1						
GB/3						
GB/8						
GB/18						

of Tu-Mo and Jen-Mo, these two categories have been left out so that the practical purpose of the charts will not be confused. This purpose is that, given two or more meridians are disordered, which single point is to be treated?

| out of order | | | | | | Point for insertion |
| YANG | | | | | | |
LI	TW	SI	B	GB	S	
			+		+	S/1
		+			+	S/6
+	+			+	+	S/12
+	+	+		+		SI/12
	+	+				SI/18
		+	+	+	+	B/1
			+	+		B/11
			+	+		B/33
	+	+		+		GB/1
+	+			+	+	GB/3
			+	+		GB/8
	+		+	+		GB/18

Points for insertion	Meridians					
	YIN					
	H	P	Lu	Lv	SP	K
20/GB						
21/GB						
24/GB					+	
13/TM						
22/TM						
25/TM						
3/JM				+	+	+
4/JM				+	+	+
10/JM			+		+	
12/JM			+			
13/JM						
17/JM	+			+	+	
6/SP				+	+	+
25/K		+		+		+
1/P		+		+		
13/Lv				+		
14/Lv				+	+	

54

out of order						Point for insertion
YANG						
LI	TW	SI	B	GB	S	
	+			+		20/GB
	+			+	+	21/GB
				+		24/GB
+	+	+	+	+	+	13/TM
	+			+		22/TM
+					+	25/TM
+	+	+	+	+	+	3/JM
						4/JM
					+	10/JM
			+		+	12/JM
		+			+	13/JM
	+	+				17/JM
						6/SP
						25/K
	+			+		1/P
				+		13/Lv
						14/Lv

CHAPTER FIVE

THE REGULATION OF ENERGY

The points of common action are used to regulate in a given and common direction (tonic or dispersive) the energy of several meridians which together present the same fault of deficiency or excess.

But more often than not examination of the pulses reveals a deficiency of energy in one or more meridians at the same time as an excess in one or more others.

That is where the technique of regulation comes in; this consists in connecting the meridians held to be strong with those which are weaker.

Acupuncture handles the energy within the body, and not that between the body and the outside world. The energy of the internal circuit of the organism can neither be created nor got rid of (at least, not to any great extent): it can only be moved from one place to another. When a meridian is strong, one must look for a weaker meridian into which its excess energy can be sent; if it is weak, one must find a stronger meridian to draw upon. This problem of regulation is solved by the intermeridional connections which their control points govern. These connections can be summarized in the five commandments of acupuncture. Three of these rules relate to the circuit of the circulation of energy; the others concern the locations of the radial pulses.

Rule 1 MOTHER-SON
Any stimulation applied by way of tonification or dispersion produces repercussions in the same direction on the meridian which precedes the one treated and on the one which follows them in the main circulation, when their pulses have comparable values.

Rule 2 LEU-TSHEU
Leu means *flow*, Tsheu, *block*. When a deficient meridian succeeds a meridian in excess, the insertion of a gold needle at the point of entry of the deficient meridian makes the energy of the strong meridian flow into the weak one. A needle inserted at the point of exit blocks the flow of energy. If the originally deficient meridian, which is now filled by that operation, is in its turn stronger than the one that follows it, the same operation is repeated on the latter, and so on:one produces flow, then one blocks. (R. Casez in *Bulletin de la Société d'Acupuncture*, No. 22, 4th Quarter, 1956.)

Rule 3 MIDDAY-MIDNIGHT
A stimulus applied to the tonification, dispersion, or Luo points of a meridian causes an inverse reaction in that which is diametrically opposed to it in the circuit of the circulation of energy. Thus, to tonify the stomach disperses the pericardium.

Rule 4 HUSBAND-WIFE
The tonic or dispersive stimulation of a meridian has a contrary action in that which is symmetrically opposed to it in the table of pulses: to disperse husband SI strengthens wife LI.

Rule 5 PAIRED MERIDIANS

When the energy level of two meridians which are superimposed in the table of pulses is different, a stimulus applied to the Luo point of one of them produces the opposite effect on the other.

Careful study and application of these rules after an adequate appraisement of the pulse levels enable a good many points to be eliminated because of their reciprocal action. This permits the circulation of energy to be regulated with a minimum of needles. Then come the specialized points and, if necessary, the sub-branch points which will thus form the completion of an effective and lasting treatment.

TREATMENT CARD

Name:				Date:

	Pulses Chart			Treatment
Right		Left		
YIN	YANG	YANG	YIN	
p	tw	b	k	
sp	s	gb	lv	
lu	li	si	h	

Circuit of Circulation

THE TECHNIQUE OF REGULATION

After a brief preliminary feeling of the pulsations of both radial arteries, which gives a general idea of the patient's energy, each of the six pulses is appraised with care and rated from 0 to 5, as has been explained on page 17. The values are recorded in the corresponding boxes of the pulses chart and in those of the inner ring of the main circulation circuit appearing on the treatment card, a sample of which is given on page 59.

In this way, it is possible to depict the disturbances in the circulation of energy, the meridians in which the latter is in excess or in shortage, and, as a result, the rule or rules of common action to be brought into play. When several meridians together present the same shortcoming, whether lack or excess, the table of the ordinary centre-reunion points can be of great assistance by enabling them all to be regulated with a single needle.

It is only after the regulation is completed and checked by taking the pulses again that it will be possible to bring into play the specialized point and any sub-branch points which will round off the treatment.

CONCLUSION

Casting an eye over this simple handbook, the novice and the layman will certainly be surprised and disappointed not to discover in it a formula, prescription or miracle points for curing at a stroke any disease whatever. Such is not the aim, although there are many works written with that intention.

The intention has been to seek out the 'root of the ill' and eradicate it. As G. Soulié de Morant says, the real origin of disease is, for the Chinese, the obstacle which crops up in the circulation of energy and disturbs its free passage in the meridians, the ultimate role of acupuncture being to raise this obstacle by stimulating the appropriate point.

And complete knowledge of the control points of the meridians and the points of common action, as well as the rules of reciprocal action, is indispensable for achieving regulation of the circuit of energy with a minimum of needles, thus tending towards the master teacher's ideal of the single needle.

Today the discovery of a multitude of new points (extraneous points, 'neo-acupuncture' points), which are added to the non-meridian points, combined with the progress of auriculotherapy, seem to throw the whole question of the classical meridians back into the melting-pot and point to the existence of other unknown meridians. But the excellent results which can be obtained with the ancient classical theory show how effective it still is and illustrate the necessity of knowing it perfectly.

The rules of the circulation of energy are perhaps the blueprint of the cybernetic system of our organism: the pulse indicates to us the information to be disclosed to the needle, which sets the integrated circuit in motion and triggers off the reaction. But the human body still remains the 'black box'.

So let us put what we know to be the best use. Perhaps one day we shall succeed in penetrating to the heart of its mysteries!

GLOSSARY

Achilles tendon: the tendon connecting the heel with the calf.

alae: plural of *ala*, the side of the wall of the nose.

anterior: lying towards the front.

apophysis: a protuberance on a bone.

auriculotherapy: acupuncture treatment applied to the external ear.

axillary: related to the armpit.

calcaneo-cuboid: relating to the heel-bone and the bone between it and the 4th and 5th metatarsal bones (*q.v.*).

cubital: related to the cubitus (*q.v.*).

cubitus: the ulna or inner of the two bones of the forearm.

cuneiform bones: wedge-shaped bones of the foot.

cybernetic: related to the science of control and communication in animals and machines.

epicondyle: the external rounded process at the end of the humerus (*q.v.*).

epitrochlear: relating to the inner epicondyle (*q.v.*) of the humerus (*q.v.*).

fibula: the bone on the outer side of the lower leg.

humerus: the bone of the upper arm.

infero-external: lying below and on the outside.

intercostal: between the ribs.

intermeridional: among the meridians.

intermetarcarpal: lying between two of the metacarpal bones (*q.v.*).,

malleolus: the ankle-bone.

metacarpal bones: five bones of the hand between the wrist and the fingers.

metatarsal bones: the five long bones of the foot between the ankle and the toes.

metatarso-phalangeal: relating to the joint between the metatarsal bones (*q.v.*) and the phalanges (*q.v.*).

olecranon: the bony prominence at the elbow.

paravertebral: situated alongside the spinal column.

pericardium: the membranous sac enclosing the heart.

phalanges: plural of *phalanx*, a finger or toe bone.

pisiform bone: a small pea-shaped bone in the wrist.

posterior: lying towards the back.

proximal: situated towards the centre of the body.

pubis: the bone at the front of the pelvis.

radius: the outer of the two bones of the forearm.

sacral fossa: a shallow depression in the sacrum (*q.v.*).

scaphoid bone: a boat-shaped bone at the front of the ankle.

spinous: pointed; pointing backwards.

sternum: the breast-bone.

styloid: long and tapered (bone).

tarso-metatarsal: involving the ankle-bones and those between the ankle and toes.

tibia: the shin-bone.

tragus: the prominence at the front of the entrance to the external ear.

tubercle: a small rounded projection on a bone.

unciform bone: a hook-shaped bone in the hand.

xiphoid appendage: the sword-shaped process at the lower end of the breast-bone.

zygoma: the bony arch on each side of the skull.